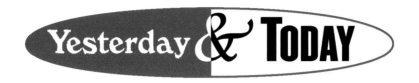

MEDICINE

Gail B. Stewart

BLACKBIRCH®
PRESS

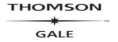

San Diego • Detroit • New York • San Francisco • Cleveland • New Haven, Conn. • Waterville, Maine • London • Munich

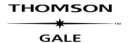

For more information, contact
The Gale Group, Inc.
27500 Drake Rd.
Farmington Hills, MI 48331-3535
Or you can visit our Internet site at http://www.gale.com

Picture Credits
Cover: © Art Today, Inc. (top), COREL Corporation (bottom)
AP/Wide World Photos, 27 (inset), 29
© Archivo Iconografico, S.A./CORBIS, 4 (top), 8
© Art Today, Inc., 17 (top), 18
© Bettmann/CORBIS, 10, 11, 12, 15, 19, 21, 22, 25, 26, 28
CDC/Dr. Fred Murphy, Sylvia Whitfield, 12 (bottom right)
© CORBIS, 20
© COREL Corporation, 12 (bottom left)
© Vo Trung Du/CORBIS SYGMA, 17
© Dr. Michael Echols, 16 (inset)
© Image Club, 9 (both)
© Laurent/Lae./American Hospital of Paris/Photo Researchers, Inc., 23
© Mary Evans Picture Library, 7
© Mediscan/Visuals Unlimited, 24
© Bazuki Muhammad/Reuters, 17 (bottom)
© North Wind Picture Archives, 4, 5 (bottom), 14
© PhotoDisc, 12 (top both), 25 (inset), 27, 31
© Reunion des Musees Nationaux/Art Resource, NY, 6, 16 (bottom)

LIBRARY OF CONGRESS CATALOGING-IN-PUBLICATION DATA

Stewart, Gail B., 1949–
  Medicine / Gail B. Stewart
      v. cm. — (Yesterday and today)
Contents: Medicine and religion—Medicine becomes a science—Understanding human anatomy—Improving surgery—Viewing the invisible—Protection from a dreaded disease—Tools that help doctors understand the body—Keeping infections at bay—Seeing inside the human body—Making surgery safer—The miracle drug—Treating mental illness with medicine—Spare parts—Gene therapy.
   ISBN 1-56711-833-X
   1. Medicine—Juvenile Literature. [1. Medicine.] I. Title. II. Series.

R129.S745 2004
610—dc21   2003023475

Table of Contents

Medicine and Religion

FAST FACT

Modern scientists know that prehistoric people in Australia chewed eucalyptus leaves when they had a fever or a bad cold. Eucalyptus is still used in many modern over-the-counter cold remedies.

Leaders of prehistoric communities sometimes danced or chanted prayers to drive away the evil spirits that were thought to cause sickness.

There are no records of medicine or doctors from prehistoric times. Even so, scientists know that people who lived more than ten thousand years ago got sick, just as they do today. In those days, however, people did not understand why they got rashes, high fevers, or stomachaches. They did not know how the organs, muscles, and bones of the body worked, so they were unable to explain diseases in a scientific way. Instead, prehistoric people used religion to explain disease. They believed that when they did something wrong, evil spirits would make them sick.

Each prehistoric community had a religious leader, or shaman. The shaman was thought to have magical powers and ways of driving evil spirits away. Sometimes the shaman would dance

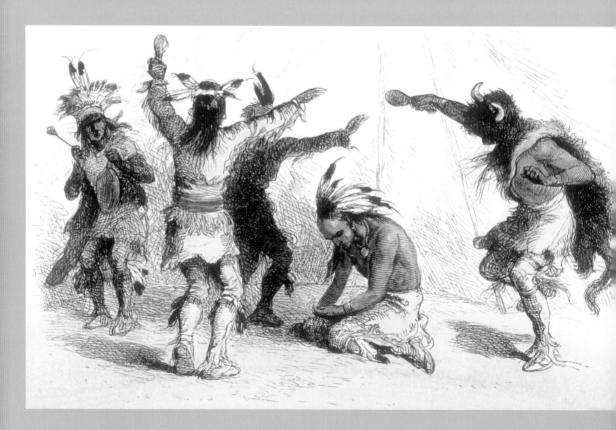

or recite special prayers to help a sick person get well. Other times, a shaman would offer special medicines made from plants. Berries from the juniper tree, for example, could help cure a bad cough. The bark from a willow tree could help a person get rid of a headache. Catnip could help someone whose stomach was upset.

Sometimes a shaman would perform surgery to rid the body of evil spirits. One of the earliest surgeries was trepanning, or drilling a hole in the skull of a person who was mentally ill or who had seizures. Shamans believed that the hole allowed evil spirits a chance to leave the body quickly. Many trepanned skulls have been found that date back more than ten thousand years. The prehistoric surgery was done with a sharp knife or piece of volcanic rock that was as sharp as glass. After the hole was made, the shaman usually covered it with a rock or shell so it could heal.

Although these prehistoric healers did not have any scientific training, they were able to help their patients. Because many of the things they did to heal their patients were successful, civilizations that came after them followed some of the same procedures.

FAST FACT

Though the technique of trepanning was developed tens of thousands of years ago, it was used by some doctors until the nineteenth century. These later doctors did not drill holes in the skull to release evil spirits, but to relieve pressure on a patient's brain.

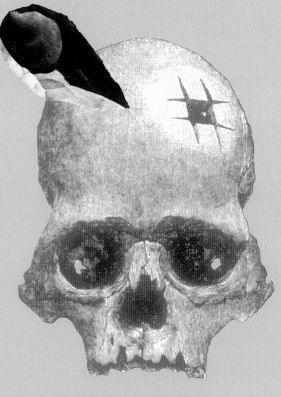

To cure the mentally ill, shamans drilled a hole in the skull to allow evil spirits to leave the patient's body. Rocks were carved into sharp knives to perform prehistoric surgery.

Prehistory

500 B.C.

100 B.C.

A.D. 100

200

500

1000

1200

1300

1400

1500

1600

1700

1800

1900

2000

2100

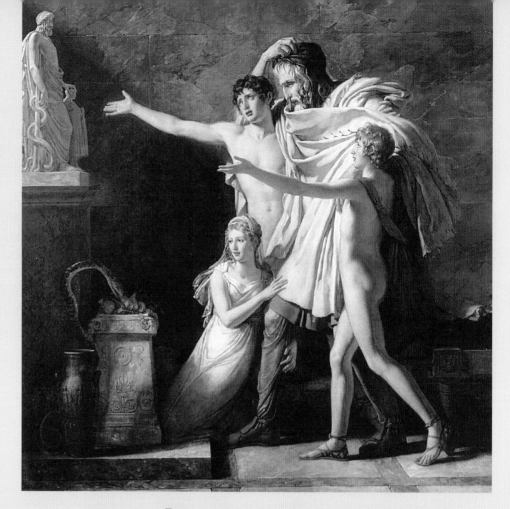

In ancient Greece, the sick often visited temples of Asklepios, the god of healing, to ask for help.

Medicine Becomes a Science

During the time of the great ancient civilizations of Egypt and Greece, medicine was still cloaked in religious mystery. Disease was still considered a punishment by the gods. In ancient Egypt, sick people sought help from priests and fortune-tellers, as well as from physicians, or healers. In ancient Greece, there were temples dedicated to Asklepios, who was believed to be the god of healing. The sick visited those temples to ask Asklepios for help.

In the fifth century B.C., however, a Greek physician named Hippocrates suggested that disease was not caused by angry gods or evil spirits. Instead, he insisted that disease was the result of physical causes. Hippocrates said that physicians could cure sick people without consulting fortune-tellers or priests. He believed that medicine was a science. If physicians looked hard enough, he said, they could find the natural cause of the illness within the patient's body.

Hippocrates was the first person to keep case histories of his patients. He wrote down details about each patient's disease. He listed each one's symptoms as well as what treatments were tried. He also described whether or not the treatments were successful.

Between A.D. 100 and 200, another Greek physician named Claudius Galen added to Hippocrates' idea that medicine was a science. Galen dissected, or cut up, dead animals and recorded his observations. Based on his dissections of apes, oxen, and pigs, Galen developed theories on the way the body works. He collected his observations in a book called *Medical Knowledge by Dissection*, written around A.D. 185. Galen's book was used as a textbook for doctors for hundreds of years.

Claudius Galen, depicted here as he treats a wounded gladiator, shared Hippocrates' view that medicine is a science and that diseases have physical causes.

The Prince of Doctors

Because of his books and his skill as a doctor, Galen was often referred to as "the Prince of Doctors." He traveled to Rome and was given the honor of being the royal physician to Emperor Marcus Aurelius.

Prehistory —

500 B.C. —

100 B.C. —

A.D. 100 —

200 —

500 —

1000 —

1200 —

1300 —

1400 —

1500 —

1600 —

1700 —

1800 —

1900 —

2000 —

2100 —

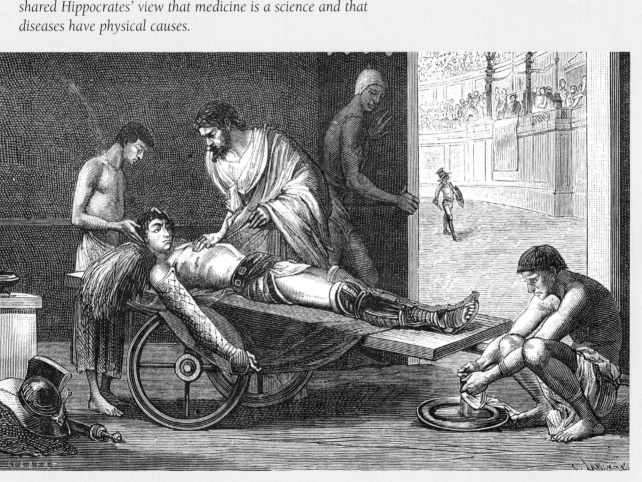

Understanding Human Anatomy

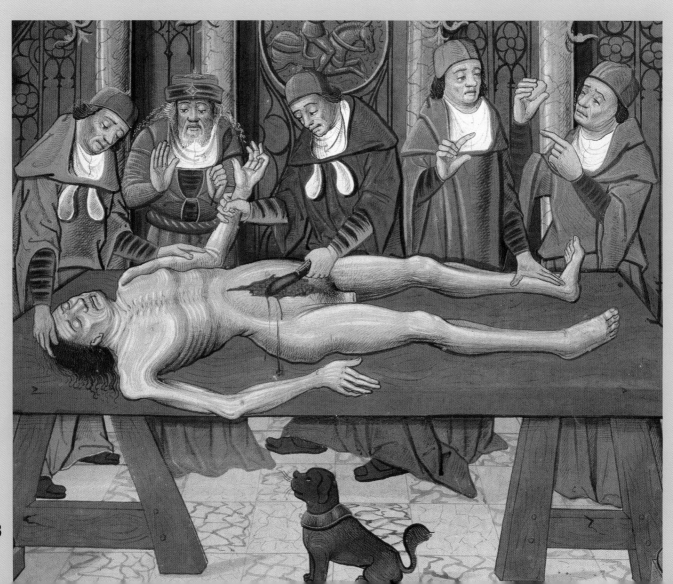

Leonardo da Vinci

Many religious leaders forbade human dissection until the late fifteenth century, when they allowed only the bodies of hanged criminals to be dissected.

For many years, medical students could learn about the human body only by studying the bodies of dead animals. Human dissection was forbidden by many religious leaders. They insisted that human dissection might keep the dead person from going to heaven. In 1482, the church agreed to allow some dissections, but only of the bodies of criminals who had been hanged.

Some of the early dissections were performed about 1510 by Leonardo da Vinci, an Italian artist and scientist. He recorded what he saw in more than 750 detailed drawings. These drawings

Circulation

Some scientists used the new knowledge of anatomy to discover more about how the body works. For example, in 1618, an English physician named William Harvey studied the pulsing arteries in the body. He noted that their pulsing was the same rhythm of the beating heart. Harvey discovered that the heart is actually a muscle that pumps blood throughout the body.

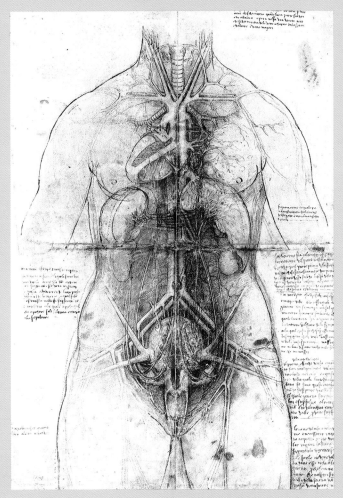

Leonardo da Vinci performed some of the earliest human dissections and used what he saw to draw detailed illustrations of the human body.

showed the placement of various muscles and organs of the human body for the first time.

Not long afterward, a Belgian physician named Andreas Vesalius began his own dissections—and made a startling discovery. Vesalius found that some of the teachings of Galen were incorrect. For instance, from his study of monkeys, Galen had taught that the heart was in the center of the chest. In humans, Vesalius noted, the heart was not in the exact center of the chest, but on the left side.

Vesalius published a book in 1543 called *The Fabric of the Human Body*. It included three hundred illustrations of the skeleton, muscles, and organs. Many church leaders were angry that Vesalius had found mistakes in Galen's work. They did not want to see such ancient wisdom challenged. Even so, Vesalius's book won the respect of physicians in Europe. It gradually replaced Galen's text as the one used to teach medical students.

Prehistory

500 B.C.

100 B.C.

A.D. 100

200

500

1000

1200

1300

1400

1500

1600

1700

1800

1900

2000

2100

In the 1500s, barbers performed most simple surgery. They pulled teeth and bandaged wounds in addition to giving haircuts. Barbers also used leeches to bleed, or drain blood from, patients who were sick. It was thought that some disease was caused by having too much blood in the body.

Improving Surgery

Although doctors had learned a great deal about the body by the 1500s, they rarely performed surgery. Operations that are common today, such as having one's tonsils or appendix removed, were almost never done. The main reason was the high risk of infection from surgical wounds. Historians estimate that infection killed almost 90 percent of surgical patients. Sometimes doctors had no choice but to perform surgery, however. When a soldier was shot by an arrow or stabbed by a sword in battle, doctors had to operate. But the chances of survival were slim.

One young surgeon, Ambroise Paré, served in the French army as a doctor in 1529, when guns were still a new weapon. Doctors struggled with the problem of how to remove bullets from wounded soldiers and repair damage to tissue and muscle. Like all wounds, gunshot

French army doctor Ambroise Paré devised an effective way to treat infections in soldiers with gunshot wounds.

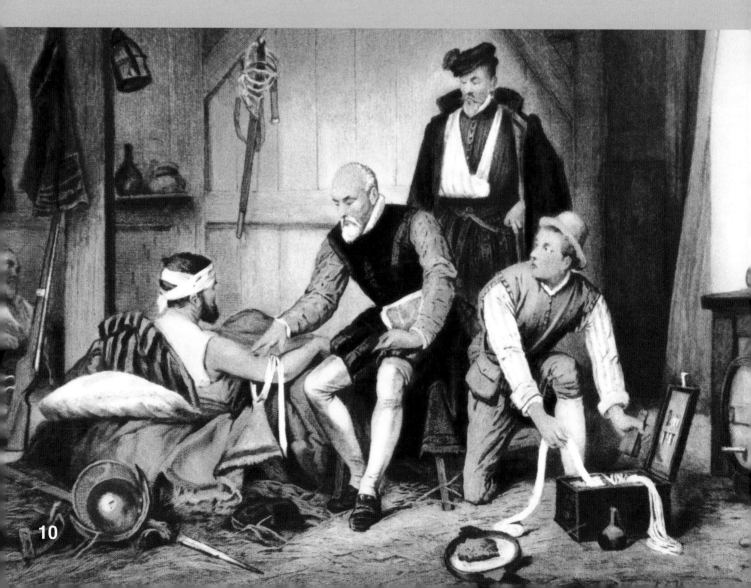

Until the early 1500s, surgeons applied a hot iron to seal blood vessels in order to stop the bleeding after a leg amputation (pictured).

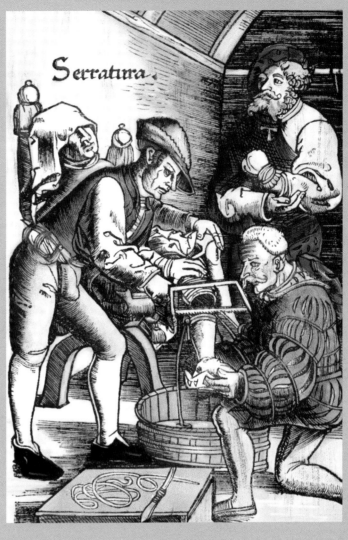

Serratura

wounds became infected very easily. Doctors in the early sixteenth century tried to prevent infection by pouring boiling oil into the wound. They believed that the hot oil would cleanse the damaged tissue.

Paré hated to hear the screams of soldiers who were being treated with burning oil or a hot iron. He wondered if there were a less painful way to close the wounds to prevent infection. One day he tried using an ointment made of egg yolk, turpentine, and rose oil— three substances found in soothing lotions of that time—to clean his patients' wounds. The ointment kept the wounds clean without causing pain.

Paré also came up with a different way to treat patients who had to have an arm or leg amputated, or removed. In those days, surgeons stopped the bleeding after amputation by sealing the blood vessels with a hot iron. This, too, was agonizing for patients. Paré tried his own method—he tied the bleeding veins together with thin pieces of string. The technique was successful. The string sealed the blood vessels without causing pain.

Paré wrote down his new methods of surgery in a book called *Method of Treating Wounds*, which he published in 1545. Other surgeons adopted his methods, and Paré became known as the "father of modern surgery."

FAST FACT

A person who needed surgery in the sixteenth century did not have drugs to dull the pain. Instead, the doctor would offer his patient a large drink of whiskey before the surgery began.

Prehistory

500 B.C.

100 B.C.

A.D. 100

200

500

1000

1200

1300

1400

1500

1600

1700

1800

1900

2000

2100

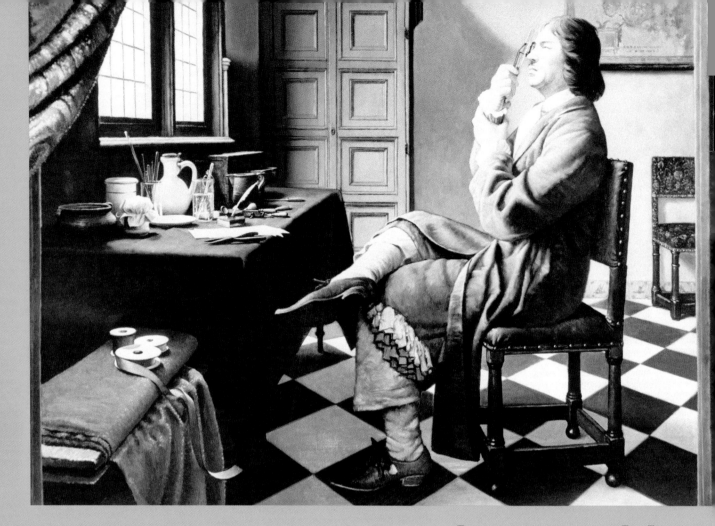

Antoni van Leeuwenhoek designed powerful microscopes that allowed him to see tiny organisms, which he drew and showed to other scientists.

Viewing the Invisible

While new surgical techniques helped doctors treat sick or wounded patients, there were still a great many things doctors did not know. For instance, doctors did not understand the cause of disease, for they had never seen germs or viruses. They were limited by what they could see with their own eyes.

In 1590, however, that began to change. A Dutch eyeglass maker named Zacharias Janssen invented a microscope with two pieces of curved glass, called lenses. Using Janssen's new microscope, a person could magnify an object nine or ten times. While this was not enough to see germs, it allowed people to see things they had never imagined. More scientists began to work with lenses to improve on Janssen's microscope.

An Englishman named Robert Hooke could magnify objects thirty times with his microscope. In the 1660s, Hooke made dozens of drawings of the details of a flea, a snowflake, and a piece of cork. He also became the first person to identify cells under his microscope.

No one made a bigger contribution to microscope research, however, than a Dutch cloth maker named Antoni van Leeuwenhoek. He made his own lenses, and they were so well made that his microscopes could magnify things up to three hundred times. It was not simply the quality of his microscopes that was important—it was the things he chose to look at. Leeuwenhoek looked at rainwater and saw tiny animals swimming in it. He scraped a little white matter from his front teeth and saw the animals there, too.

Leeuwenhoek drew pictures of the things he saw and shared them with a group of scientists called the Royal Society. They published his drawings for others to see. Over the next century, his findings led scientists to more exploration with microscopes. Some wondered about the tiny animals swimming in drops of rainwater, or in their own mouths. Eventually, Leeuwenhoek's discovery led scientists to realize that these tiny animals were responsible for disease and infection in human beings.

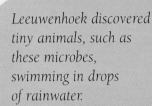

Leeuwenhoek discovered tiny animals, such as these microbes, swimming in drops of rainwater.

Microscopes enabled Robert Hooke to see the details of a piece of cork (left) in the 1660s and later scientists to discover that organisms like smallpox cells (right) cause disease.

Prehistory

500 B.C.

100 B.C.

A.D. 100

200

500

1000

1200

1300

1400

1500

1600

1700

1800

1900

2000

2100

13

Protection from a Dreaded Disease

While some physicians speculated on the microscopic causes of disease, others were fighting a losing battle against one of the most feared diseases in history—smallpox. The first written account of a smallpox epidemic was by a physician in Persia (present-day Iran) in the year A.D. 845. He described victims as having high fevers followed by severe raised sores on their skin. Smallpox was highly contagious. It often spread quickly through entire cities and towns, killing thousands at a time. One-third of all who caught smallpox died. Those who survived were often blind and scarred from the disease.

In the late 1700s, an English doctor named Edward Jenner tried to find a way to protect people from the disease. Jenner

Edward Jenner discovered a vaccine for smallpox in the late 1700s and within two hundred years, scientists declared that one of the most feared diseases in the world was dead.

14

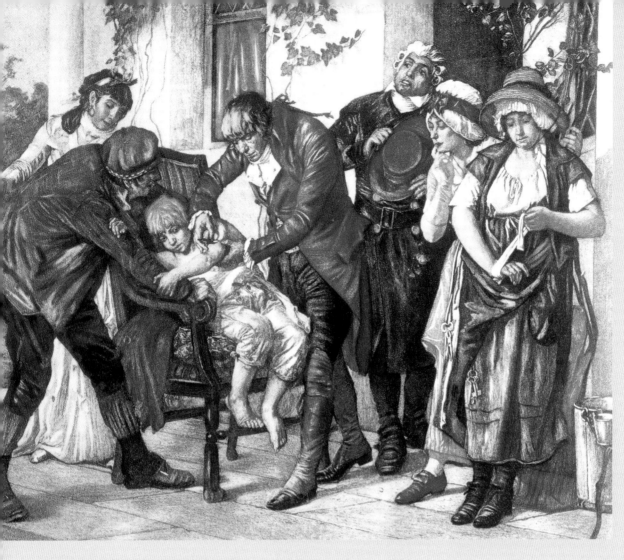

Prehistory —

500 B.C. —

100 B.C. —

A.D. 100 —

200 —

500 —

1000 —

1200 —

1300 —

1400 —

1500 —

1600 —

1700 —

1800 —

1900 —

2000 —

2100 —

had heard that dairymaids never caught smallpox. He wondered if that was because the young women often caught cowpox—a disease related to smallpox—from the cows they milked. Cowpox, while dangerous to cows, was not harmful at all to humans. Usually, it caused only a few skin sores, which gradually went away.

Jenner tested his theory by scratching pus from the sores of a girl with cowpox into the arm of an eight-year-old boy named James. After two weeks, he deliberately injected James with smallpox, but James did not develop the disease. Jenner concluded that the tiny amount of cowpox germs had kept James from getting smallpox. Others whom he infected with bits of cowpox pus also stayed smallpox-free. Although a cure for the disease had not been found, it was now possible to protect people from it.

In 1796, Jenner vaccinated an eight-year-old boy against smallpox by using cowpox pus from the hand of a dairymaid.

Tools That Help Doctors Understand the Body

As the science of medicine grew, doctors concentrated on preventing disease. One way to do that was to keep track of the vital signs that indicate health or sickness. One sign is the sound of a healthy heart and lungs. Until the nineteenth century, doctors had to put their ear to a patient's chest to listen to breathing sounds. In 1816, however, a young French doctor named René Laënnec created an instrument known as the stethoscope. It helped doctors hear much better.

The first stethoscope was a wooden cylinder about nine inches long. The doctor would put his ear to one end and place the other on the patient's chest. Doctors could detect irregular heartbeats through Laënnec's

After René Laënnec (center) invented the stethoscope (inset), doctors could easily listen to a patient's heart and lungs.

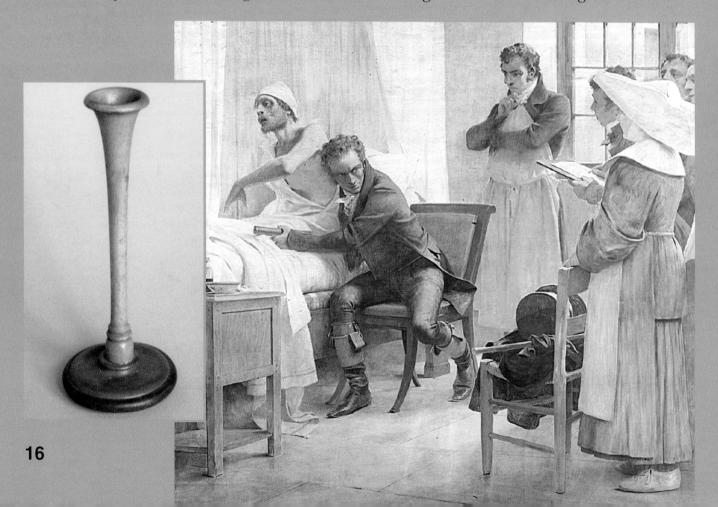

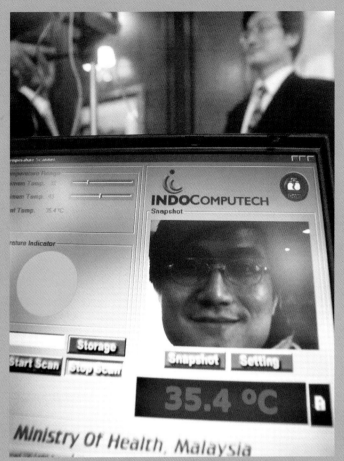

Today, an electronic health monitor can measure a person's vital signs and send the data through a computer.

Prehistory —

500 B.C. —

100 B.C. —

A.D. 100 —

200 —

500 —

1000 —

1200 —

1300 —

1400 —

1500 —

1600 —

1700 —

1800 —

1900 —

2000 —

2100 —

stethoscope. They could also diagnose a patient whose lungs were affected by pneumonia or other diseases.

Another vital measurement is the body's temperature. Before the medical thermometer, doctors felt a patient's forehead to check for a fever. Various types of thermometers had been in use since the late sixteenth century. These were too large and inaccurate, however, to determine an exact body temperature. In 1866, Thomas Allbutt invented the first medical thermometer. It was small—only six inches long —and could easily fit in a patient's mouth.

With tools such as these, doctors could measure the changes in the body that certain diseases caused, such as rapid heartbeat or elevated temperature. This ability made it easier for doctors to give each patient a more accurate diagnosis, too.

Thermometers

While some doctors still use a thermometer very much like the one invented in 1866, there have been some modern improvements. Some are plastic, which are cheaper to produce and can be thrown away after a single use. Others are plastic strips that do not need to go in a patient's mouth. Instead, they are pressed to the forehead and give a digital display.

Keeping Infections at Bay

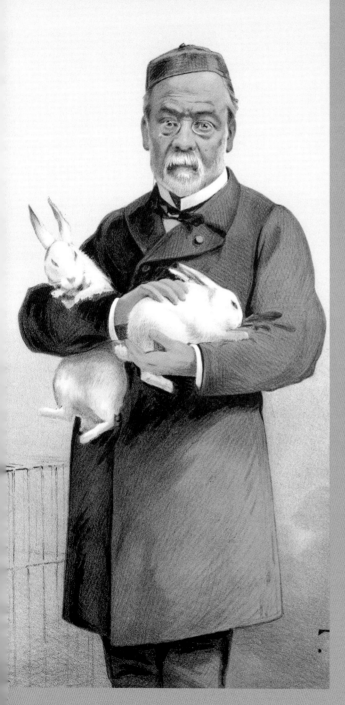

French scientist Louis Pasteur suggested that microorganisms called germs could cause diseases in humans and animals.

A French scientist named Louis Pasteur was asked to look into a problem that was puzzling local wine-makers. Some of their wine had a bitter taste, and they had no explanation. Pasteur looked at samples of the wine under his microscope and saw that the bitter wine had many tiny germs in it. He declared that the germs were responsible for the bad taste. He also suggested that tiny germs could harm people and animals, too. Pasteur and other scientists identified germs that caused several diseases.

British surgeon Joseph Lister was intrigued by Pasteur's discoveries. Like many other doctors of his day, Lister was discouraged by the large number of patients who died of infections after surgery. He wondered if the infections could be caused by microscopic germs. To test his theory, he used a chemical called carbolic acid to kill germs in his patients' surgical wounds. Lister also used carbolic acid to clean his hands and surgical instruments before he operated. He even sprayed a mist of carbolic acid in the room while he operated. Lister was pleased by the results, for his patients suffered from far fewer infections.

FAST FACT

Louis Pasteur found that one way to kill harmful bacteria in milk was to heat it to exactly 135 degrees Fahrenheit. Today, the process of heating milk to destroy bacteria is called pasteurization, in his honor.

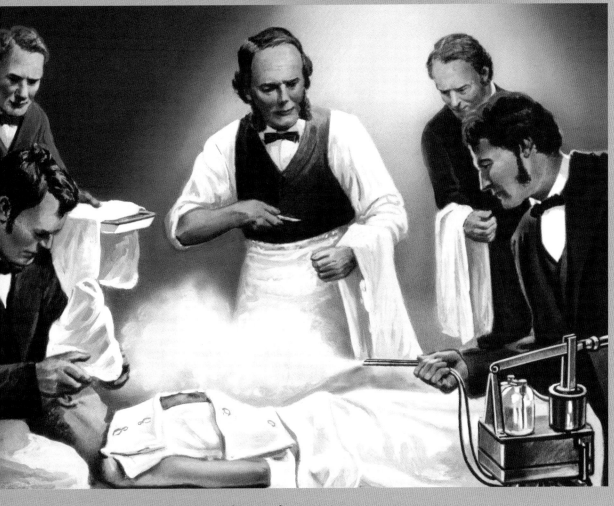

Joseph Lister's patients developed fewer infections when he began to use carbolic acid to clean wounds, his hands, and surgical instruments.

Johnson & Johnson, an American manufacturer of surgical supplies, believed that bandages and other dressings for wounds could be sterilized in the factory. In 1886, the company introduced bandages that had been treated with antiseptic, or germ-killing, chemicals. Each bandage was individually wrapped so that a surgeon would know it was free of germs.

The growing attention to cleanliness as a way to prevent germs from spreading continued. As a result, patients began to recover more quickly from disease and injury.

FAST FACT

Until Joseph Lister's day, it was common for doctors to go from one patient to the next without washing their hands. After it was proved that germs cause infection, hand washing became a must for doctors and nurses.

Prehistory —

500 B.C. —

100 B.C. —

A.D. 100 —

200 —

500 —

1000 —

1200 —

1300 —

1400 —

1500 —

1600 —

1700 —

1800 —

1900 —

2000 —

2100 —

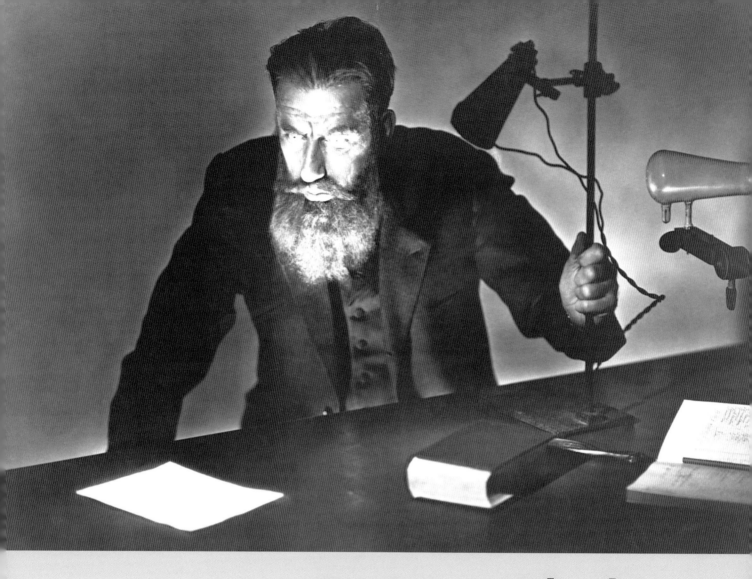

Seeing Inside the Human Body

The Fluoroscope

In 1896, the famous American inventor Thomas A. Edison invented a special machine called a fluoroscope, with which doctors could view X-ray photographs. Its screen makes the X-ray image glow, which in turn makes it easier to see. Even though he knew that once his invention was patented it could make a lot of money, Edison chose not to apply for a patent for the fluoroscope. He knew that the patent process could take more than a year, and he believed doctors should not have to wait that long to help their sick patients.

By the end of the nineteenth century, doctors knew more about the health of their patients than ever before. They noted vital signs such as heartbeat and temperature, and they understood that changes in those signs could be indications of disease. There were still some things, however, that doctors could not know without performing surgery to see inside the body. For example, a doctor who needed to operate on a wounded soldier could not be sure where the bullet was until he began to cut.

In 1895, however, a German scientist made an exciting new discovery that provided a wealth of information to doctors. The scientist, Wilhelm Röntgen, made his

Prehistory ——

500 B.C. ——

100 B.C. ——

A.D. 100 ——

200 ——

500 ——

1000 ——

1200 ——

1300 ——

1400 ——

1500 ——

1600 ——

1700 ——

1800 ——

1900 ——

2000 ——

2100 ——

Opposite: German scientist Wilhelm Röntgen discovered X-rays by accident in 1895. His discovery allowed doctors to see inside their patients' bodies.

discovery by accident. He was experimenting with electric currents and a glass tube. Each time he sent the electric current through the glass, a piece of special photographic paper lying on a table nearby would change. It was as if light had hit the paper, which it had not. Röntgen realized that invisible rays were affecting the paper. He called them "X-rays," because "x" is a mathematical symbol for "unknown."

Röntgen found that X-rays could penetrate many materials that light rays cannot, such as skin. However, harder material, such as bone, blocked the X-rays. Röntgen developed a way to take photographs of the body using X-rays. One of the first pictures he took showed the bones in his wife's hand in remarkable detail. Other scientists did their own experiments with X-rays. Soon the process became an important tool for doctors to use when examining their patients.

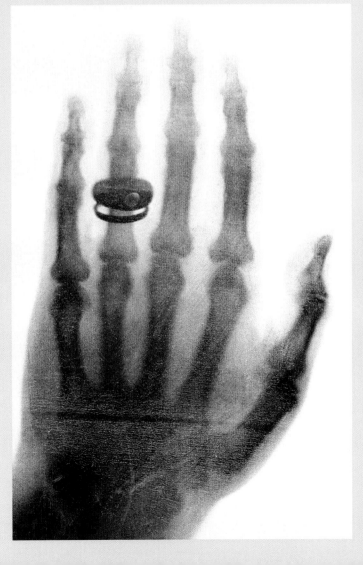

Right: One of the first X-rays Röntgen took was of the bones in his wife's hand.

21

Making Surgery Safer

Several exciting advances in medicine in the early 1900s made surgery safer than ever before. One was the discovery that all human blood is not the same. Since the seventeenth century, doctors had been able to give blood transfusions, or transfer blood to a patient from an outside source. The new blood, however, often caused patients to become very ill—sometimes fatally so.

In 1902, an Austrian doctor named Karl Landsteiner found that there were four types of human blood, and he called them O, A, AB, and B. Each type has a different chemical makeup. Giving a transfusion of type A blood to a person whose blood type was B, for instance, was highly dangerous. From that point on, surgeons were careful to match blood types of patients to blood donors.

Karl Landsteiner discovered that there are four types of human blood.

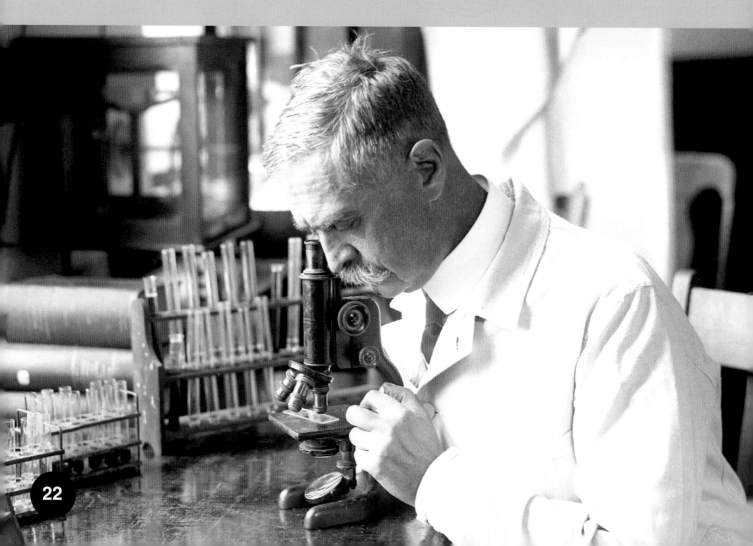

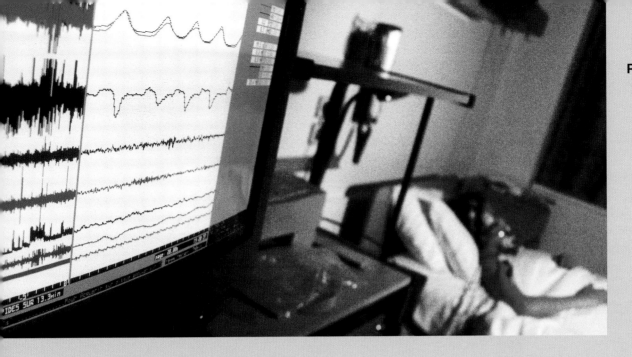

Doctors use an EEG to measure electrical currents when they diagnose injuries and diseases in the brain.

Another important advance for doctors was the invention of the electrocardiograph, commonly called the EKG. An Italian scientist, Carlo Matteucci, had shown in 1830 that every time the heart beats, it generates a pulse of electricity. In 1903, a Dutch scientist named Willem Einthoven invented a machine that could monitor those pulses and display each beat of a patient's heart on a photographic plate.

Einthoven's machine allowed doctors to see whether a patient's heartbeat was normal or abnormal. Over time the information helped doctors diagnose various types of heart trouble early. This gave patients a better chance of recovery from heart disease.

In 1924, Einthoven's heart monitor inspired a German doctor named Hans Berger to measure brain activity in the same way. He attached thin wires to the brains of patients who were having brain surgery. Berger attached the wires to a machine that could record and display the electrical currents. Over several years, Berger was able to make the wires, called electrodes, so sensitive that they could pick up electrical impulses from a patient's scalp. His machine was called the EEG, or electroencephalograph. It is used today to help doctors diagnose injuries and disease in the brain.

FAST FACT

Both the EKG and the EEG were modified over the years. Instead of only being used by doctors before surgery, either of the monitors can be used during surgery, to show the doctor if a patient is having difficulty during the operation.

Prehistory —

500 B.C. —

100 B.C. —

A.D. 100 —

200 —

500 —

1000 —

1200 —

1300 —

1400 —

1500 —

1600 —

1700 —

1800 —

1900 —

2000 —

2100 —

The Miracle Drug

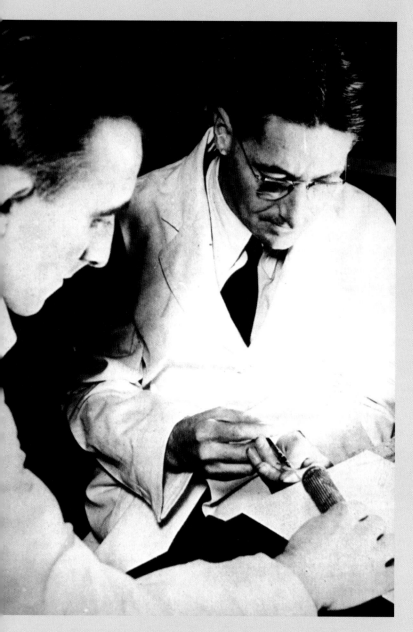

Howard Florey (pictured right), working with Ernst Chain, discovered that penicillin could kill many types of infection-causing germs while leaving healthy tissue unharmed.

Scientists in the early twentieth century understood that infections and diseases were caused by germs. It was not understood, however, how to treat a patient suffering from a serious infection. For that reason, an infection such as strep throat was often fatal, as was an infection from stepping on a rusty nail.

In 1928, a Scottish scientist named Alexander Fleming was doing research on germs. He had been studying a type of germ that causes infections in blood vessels and the heart. Fleming had samples of the germs growing in glass dishes in his laboratory.

One day he noticed a greenish mold growing in the dishes and that it had killed the germs. The mold was a rare plant called *Penicillium*. Fleming worked with the mold to try to pinpoint how it killed germs. His efforts failed, however. After several years, Fleming moved on to other projects.

In 1940, two scientists working in England, Howard Florey and Ernst Chain, took another look at Fleming's work. They found a certain chemical given off by the mold and collected it. They tested it by giving it to four mice who had been infected with a dangerous germ. The four mice quickly recovered. Florey and Chain tried their experiment on humans, and it was successful.

Soon the chemical was being called a miracle drug, for it was saving lives of soldiers battling serious infections.

Doctors were pleased that penicillin, as the drug was called, did not harm healthy tissue. It was, however, very harmful to a whole range of germs—including the ones that caused blood poisoning, strep throat, and pneumonia.

Making Penicillin

Once Florey and Chain realized that penicillin worked on humans, they took their discovery to various medical laboratories in England. Because World War II had begun, however, the companies were unwilling to spend a lot of money on the new drug. Florey and Chain visited the United States in 1941, and American companies agreed to start production of penicillin.

In 1940, Chain (pictured) and Florey continued the research on Penicillium *(inset) that had been started by Alexander Fleming in 1928.*

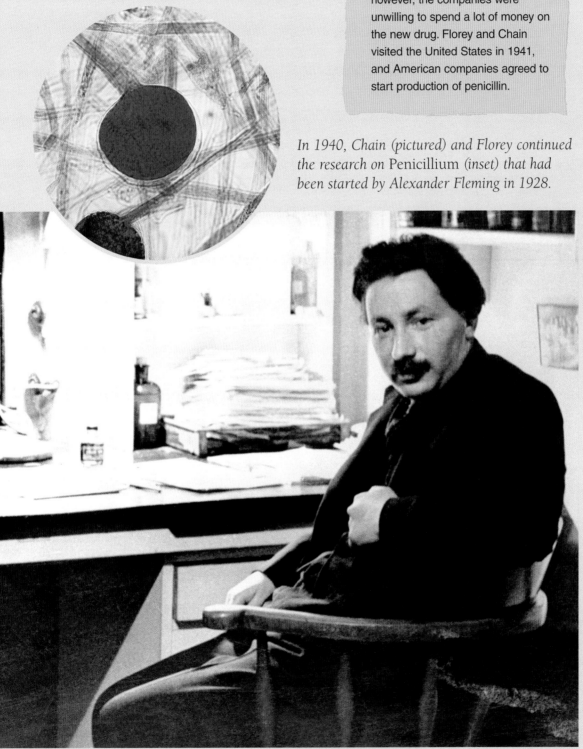

Prehistory ——

500 B.C. ——

100 B.C. ——

A.D. 100 ——

200 ——

500 ——

1000 ——

1200 ——

1300 ——

1400 ——

1500 ——

1600 ——

1700 ——

1800 ——

1900 ——

2000 ——

2100 ——

Treating Mental Illness with Medicine

Medicine for the Mind

In recent years, researchers have found that chemical imbalances may be responsible for other problems such as attention deficit disorder. This condition makes it hard for students to concentrate in school. Drugs such as Ritalin are often prescribed for children with these conditions. In 2003, it was estimated that almost 5 percent of schoolchildren take a drug like Ritalin regularly.

One branch of medicine that took a great leap forward during the twentieth century was psychiatry, the treatment of people with mental illness. Thanks to important work by Sigmund Freud in the late nineteenth century, doctors had learned that many mentally ill patients could be helped by discussing their problems and feelings with a psychiatrist.

Many other patients, however, did not benefit from such "talk therapy," as it was called. Some of these

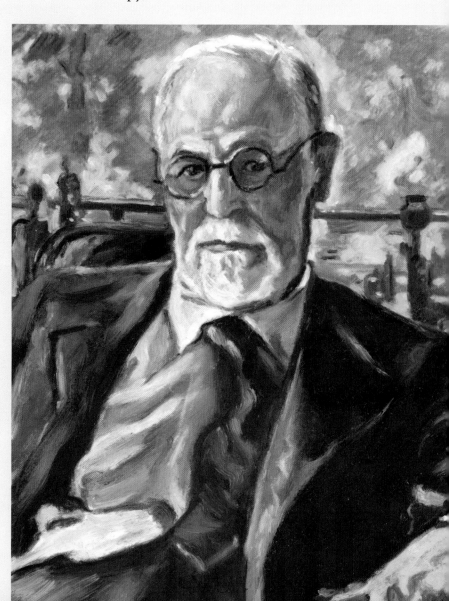

Sigmund Freud has been called the father of psychiatry because of his groundbreaking work with mentally ill patients in the late nineteenth century.

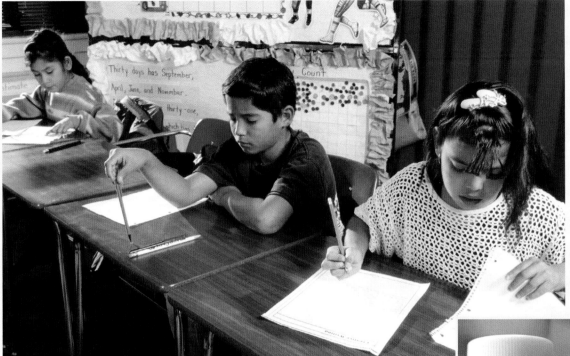

Prehistory —

500 B.C. —

100 B.C. —

A.D. 100 —

200 —

500 —

1000 —

1200 —

1300 —

1400 —

1500 —

1600 —

1700 —

1800 —

1900 —

2000 —

2100 —

patients suffered from what is now known as bipolar disorder—dramatic mood swings that range from deep depression to happy excitement. People with bipolar disorder have difficulty living normal lives because their moods are so unpredictable.

In 1949, Australian scientist John Cade did experiments to find out whether such mood swings had a chemical cause. Wondering about the effect of one chemical, lithium, on the body, he injected it into some very excitable guinea pigs. Soon the lithium caused the animals to become relaxed and sleepy. He tested lithium on himself and found that it made him relaxed, too. When he tested it on some patients with bipolar disease, their mood swings became less noticeable.

After Cade's work, researchers experimented with other chemicals that could help other mentally ill patients. In 1950, a drug called Thorazine was developed. It is helpful for people who suffer from psychotic episodes, during which they lose contact with reality. Although such drugs do not work on everyone, they have provided a way to treat the chemical imbalances that can cause mental illness.

Doctors often prescribe Ritalin (inset) to treat children with attention deficit disorder.

Spare Parts

While the methods and tools of surgery had improved over the years, doctors still faced frustrating limits. For instance, there were many patients with a kidney or other organ that was too damaged by disease or injury to repair. Some surgeons wished that transplanting an organ were possible. They wanted to be able to replace a diseased or injured organ with a healthy one.

For years, surgeons tried to transplant organs from one animal to another with little success. More often than not, the animal's body would reject an organ that was not its own. When this happened, the animal would die.

In the mid-1940s, scientists discovered that there are different tissue types just as there are different blood types. A transplant from one tissue type to another had no chance of succeeding. On the other hand, if the

In 1967, South African doctor Christiaan Barnard performed the world's first heart transplant.

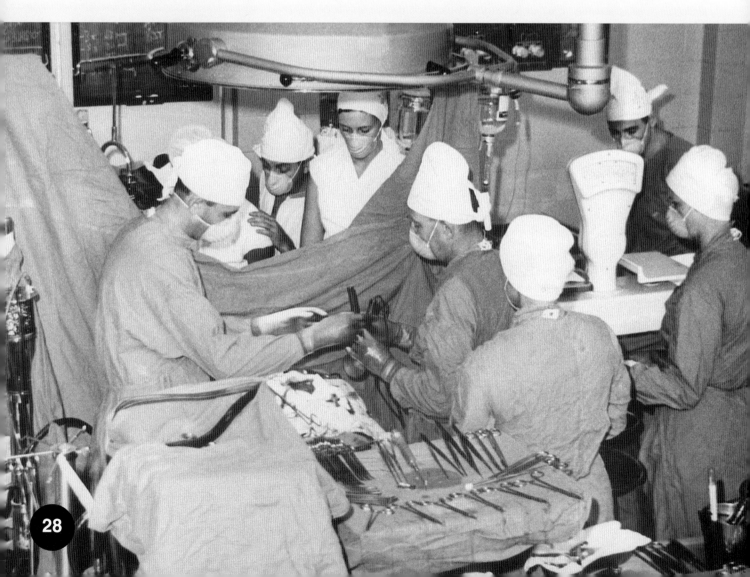

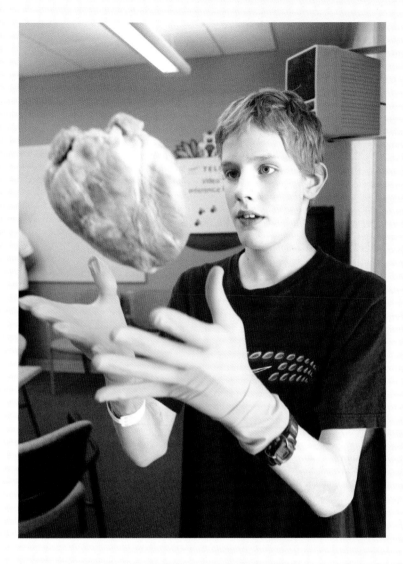

Twelve-year-old Shane Bowman played with his old heart after his 2003 heart transplant. Thousands of organs, including kidneys, lungs, livers, and corneas, are transplanted every year.

patient and the donor were related, that transplant had a better chance of success.

In 1954, the first successful human kidney transplant was performed. A patient whose two kidneys did not work had a twin who was willing to donate one kidney. Though people are born with two kidneys, they can live a normal life with just one. The patient survived and lived for seven years with the new kidney.

The first heart transplant occurred in 1967. Dr. Christiaan Barnard of South Africa transplanted the heart of a twenty-four-year-old accident victim into the body of a fifty-four-year-old man. The man lived for eighteen days before dying of pneumonia. Another transplant was done soon afterward, and this time, the patient lived for nineteen months. Within twenty years, heart transplants became more common, with more than two thousand performed each year in the United States alone.

Laser Surgery

The most common organ transplanted is the cornea, the clear covering on the colored part of the eye. One of the reasons is the development of laser surgery in the 1960s. Using a concentrated beam of light, surgeons could operate on the delicate eyeball without risk of leaving scars.

Prehistory —

500 B.C. —

100 B.C. —

A.D. 100 —

200 —

500 —

1000 —

1200 —

1300 —

1400 —

1500 —

1600 —

1700 —

1800 —

1900 —

2000 —

2100 —

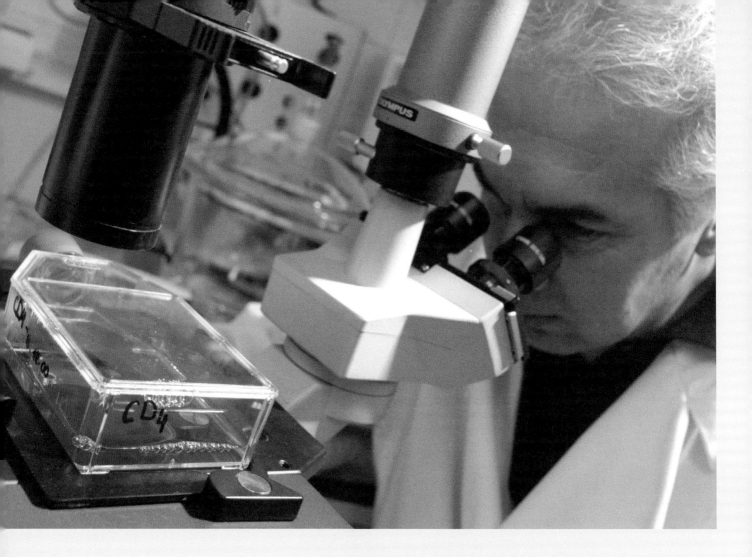

Scientists use powerful microscopes to study genes, which carry information from both parents.

Gene Therapy

As they have researched the cause of diseases over the years, scientists have learned that some are hereditary, or passed down from parents to children. Diabetes, cystic fibrosis, and some types of cancer are examples of such diseases. Genes, which can only be seen with the most powerful microscopes, carry information from both parents. Genes determine gender, height, and the color of hair and eyes. Sometimes genes may be missing or defective, and that can lead to disease.

One exciting development in medicine is gene therapy, the process of replacing a defective gene with a normal one. In 1990, U.S. doctors had a young patient whose body could not fight disease as it should. They found that a particular gene was missing from the boy's white blood cells, so they added the gene to his cells. After four months of therapy, the child was able to fight disease normally.

One of the ways scientists add genes to patients' cells is by using a virus as a delivery system. Viruses infect people by entering the nucleus, or center, of cells and inserting their own DNA. Scientists remove the disease-causing DNA from the virus and replace it with the genetic material the patient needs. The virus then inserts the needed genetic materials into the patient's cells.

Many scientists are excited about the growth of gene therapy. They see it as a way to get rid of disease even before it strikes—by eliminating the gene that causes it.

Researchers believe that gene therapy, a way to replace a defective gene with a normal one, may be a way to treat diseases or even eliminate them before they strike.

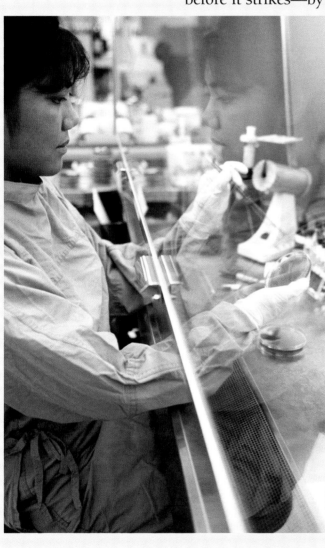

In 1997, doctors were able to isolate DNA from an unborn baby and learn whether the baby would be likely to get a certain inherited disease. Doctors say that someday they may be able to treat diseases before a baby is even born.

Others worry that gene therapy could be abused. They say that if scientists can identify particular genes, some might be tempted to design babies who are stronger, taller, or smarter. Gene therapy is one advance in medicine that has a great many risks as well as benefits.Gene therapy is the most recent link in a chain that began more than ten thousand years ago. From the time of the shamans of prehistoric societies, people have made important new medical discoveries. With each new discovery, doctors are better able to treat the sick and keep their patients healthy.

Prehistory ——

500 B.C. ——

100 B.C. ——

A.D. 100 ——

200 ——

500 ——

1000 ——

1200 ——

1300 ——

1400 ——

1500 ——

1600 ——

1700 ——

1800 ——

1900 ——

2000 ——

2100 ——

Glossary

antiseptic: Something that kills germs.

cornea: The clear, thin coating over the colored part of the eye. The cornea allows light to enter the eye.

dissection: The cutting up of a dead body as a way of studying its parts.

donor: A person who gives blood or an organ to another.

EEG: Short for electroencephalograph, the EEG is a monitor that displays the brain waves of a patient. The EEG is often used to detect diseases of the brain.

EKG: Short for electrocardiograph, an EKG is a monitor that displays the individual beats of a patient's heart.

gene: Genes are very tiny sections of DNA. Each gene determines a certain trait, such as hair color or height.

germ: A small organism that can cause disease and infection.

psychotic: Losing touch with reality. People who are psychotic usually suffer from a chemical imbalance.

shaman: A religious leader or medicine man.

smallpox: A highly contagious disease that killed millions of people through the ages. Edward Jenner discovered a vaccine for the disease in the late eighteenth century.

stethoscope: An important medical tool that allows a doctor to listen to a patient's heartbeat and breath sounds.

transfusion: The transfer of blood from the body of one person to another.

trepanning: An early form of surgery that involves drilling holes in a patient's skull.

virus: A tiny microorganism that can cause disease. Viruses are often used in gene therapy to deliver normal genes to cells.

For More Information

Books

Beverly Birch, *Pasteur's Flight Against Microbes*. Hauppauge, NY: Barron's Educational Series, 1996.

Steve Parker, *Eyewitness Science: Medicine*. London: Dorling Kindersley, 1995.

Gail Stewart, *Microscopes*. San Diego, CA: KidHaven, 2003.

Rod Storring, *A Doctor's Life: A Visual History of Doctors and Nurses Through the Ages*. New York: Dutton Children's Books, 1998.

Web Site

Human Genetics and Medical Research (www.history.nih. gov). This National Institutes of Health Web site offers eye-catching graphics with good information about early gene research, as well as gene therapy today.

Index